Sleep Affirmations

200 Phrases for a Deep and Peaceful Sleep

JENNIFER WILLIAMSON

ADAMS MEDIA

NEW YORK   LONDON   TORONTO   SYDNEY   NEW DELHI

Aadamsmedia

Adams Media
An Imprint of Simon & Schuster, Inc.
57 Littlefield Street
Avon, Massachusetts 02322

First Adams Media hardcover edition May 2018

ADAMS MEDIA and colophon are trademarks of Simon & Schuster.

For information about special discounts for bulk purchases, please contact Simon & Schuster Special Sales at 1-866-506-1949 or business@simonandschuster.com.

The Simon & Schuster Speakers Bureau can bring authors to your live event. For more information or to book an event contact the Simon & Schuster Speakers Bureau at 1-866-248-3049 or visit our website at www.simonspeakers.com.

Interior design by Colleen Cunningham
Interior images © 123RF/melpomen, Anastasiya Ramanenka, Yuliya Kulinenko; Shutterstock/Nezabudkina, suns07butterfly

Manufactured in the United States of America

10 9 8 7 6 5 4 3 2 1

Library of Congress Cataloging-in-Publication Data
Williamson, Jennifer (Jennifer Marie), 1988-, author.
Sleep affirmations / Jennifer Williamson.
Avon, Massachusetts: Adams Media, 2018.
LCCN 2017059994 (print) | LCCN 2018005283 (ebook) | ISBN 9781507207604 (hc) | ISBN 9781507207611 (ebook)
LCSH: Sleep. | Affirmations. | Mind and body. | Self-care, Health. | BISAC: SELF-HELP / Affirmations. | HEALTH & FITNESS / Sleep & Sleep Disorders. | SELF-HELP / Motivational & Inspirational.
LCC RA786 (ebook) | LCC RA786 .W55 2018 (print) | DDC 613.7/94--dc23
LC record available at https://lccn.loc.gov/2017059994

ISBN 978-1-5072-0760-4
ISBN 978-1-5072-0761-1 (ebook)

introduction

Imagine closing your eyes to the day, enjoying a good night's sleep, and waking in the morning feeling totally refreshed—mind, body, and soul. The positive sleep affirmations in this book will help you do exactly that by visualizing and inviting the restful energy that will lead you into a peaceful place.

Every declaration, whether you're speaking it out loud or thinking it to yourself, is an affirmation. "I can't sleep" and "I love sleep" are both affirmations, but the first one highlights what you don't want, while the second one asserts what you want more of. Mindful affirmations are catalysts for your desired experiences. They ferry you across the river so that you don't have to struggle upstream all on your own. The sleep affirmations in this book are carefully crafted ferryboats, intended to help you sail smoothly off to sleep.

As your affirmations become more mindful, your energy will start to resonate more deeply with the experience you want—in this case, peaceful sleep. Thankfully, you will have these two hundred soul-affirming, mind-liberating truths to support and guide you. Every affirmation is infused with quiet hope and is ready to impart the blessing of peace. Simple and insightful, these messages are easy to read and delightful to fall asleep with.

Consider this book to be your sleep companion. Consult its gentle guidance when getting ready for bed, or use it to lull yourself back to sleep in the middle of the night. Follow along in sequence, or flip to any page for your nightly passage—find what works for you. The only requirement is your willingness to receive the compassion and understanding that this book offers, through an open heart and mind.

how to use these affirmations

A quiet mind, a relaxed body, and a loving heart all work together to pave positive new pathways. Designed with your best sleep in mind, each affirmation in this book shares an easy-to-absorb, holistic message that speaks to your entire being. If you're ready for better sleep, this book can get you there.

Declare with conviction that you are ready to enjoy the peaceful sleep you've been dreaming of. Holding this book in your hands is a testament to your readiness, and the words you're reading will show you a better way. Sleep doesn't want you to struggle; sleep asks that you release the struggle. Now that you've affirmed your willingness to try something new, the fight to fall asleep is about to be transformed into something much more enjoyable.

Every page shares digestible inspiration that's both open to interpretation and rooted in wisdom. You might read the same affirmation three times, and each reading will spark new healing according to the season of life you're in. No matter what's happening in your life, the intention remains intact: you are encouraged to release the struggle, to receive the wisdom, and to enter the mindful state of peace that invites sleep.

Incorporate this book into your nightly routine, and pick it back up to help you fall asleep after waking. Though the affirmations read well in sequence, you are free to select your nightly reading by turning to a random page. To make sure these affirmations work for you, keep in mind the following suggestions:

★ Repeat one affirmation nightly. If tonight's affirmation doesn't resonate with you, or if you're not ready for the message, simply flip to the next (or another) page.

★ Take 5–10 minutes to repeat the affirmation. Take your time and let the message sink in.

★ Start by reading the words out loud, if possible. If you can't or don't want to speak the words out loud, repeat them silently to yourself.

★ Once you've placed the book back on your nightstand, let the affirmation reverberate in your mind. Loosely ponder what you remember and love most from the message—it might be one sentence or one word that sticks with you. (Many of the affirmations rhyme for easy remembering.)

★ Anchor the affirmation in your body with the mindful placement of your hands. Placing your hand on your heart or belly, holding your own hands, and cradling your face are all self-comforting mechanisms that help to establish the affirmation internally.

★ Embody the energy of the message. Say it—really experience it—with great feeling and awareness. Go beyond the words themselves and focus on the imagery they elicit.

★ When distractions arise, return to the affirmation. In this way, every disturbance becomes another chance to enjoy the affirmation's deep sentiments.

★ Affirm with sincerity and conviction. For any affirmation to work, you must believe it is true for you. This is why each message leaves room for personal exploration; no matter your beliefs, remain receptive to the energetic quality of the statement.

★ If you encounter resistance, simply be aware. In the process of using a new affirmation, old, negative, or contradicting beliefs might arise. This is not a sign of failure. Resistance to something new is natural. "I'm not worthy" and "Nothing works" are just old thoughts. Give yourself compassion, and give the new affirmation space to grow. It's all part of a larger practice.

As you practice these positive, mindful affirmations, you'll participate in the creation of what you truly want. When you relax into your creative power and embrace what's possible, sleep will become an effortless extension of your nature.

Nighttime is my time to heal.

As I hand over my thoughts to the healing night, they are carefully held for me. I entrust my worries, fears, and hurts to the universe, and all is taken care of for me. Sleep is coming to restore me back to full vitality.

My best is always good enough and
everything else is worthy of forgiveness.
I am willing to try this belief: I have done my
best. I forgive the rest. Now it's time to let go.

*I have done my best
today, and I am willing
to forgive the rest.*

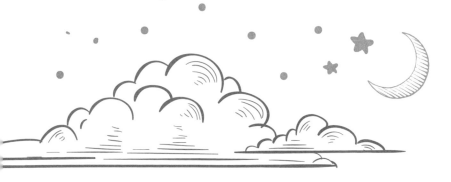

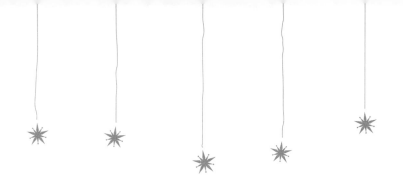

My breath is my guide
back to peace.

As I breathe in peaceful possibility, I release
any resistance to quiet in my soul. All is well and
safe here; all is right and whole. Mindful, steady
breathing carries me back home.

Sleep is calling me, and I must go.

My body listens to the whispers of night, telling me softly to be at ease. There is time enough for the day, and now it is my time to dream. The weight of the day is lifting as my thoughts are drifting toward sleep.

I Am.

Thankfully, my thoughts are not me.
I transcend all mental activity, for I am
pure consciousness. I allow thoughts to enter
and leave me with ease; I let them be carried
away like falling leaves in a gentle breeze.
I lie back and allow, because I Am.

Dear Sleep: I love you.

Thank you, pillow, for cradling my tired head.
Thank you, bed, for supporting my tired body.
Thank you, blankets, for holding my weary self.
I am grateful to be in this space,
held in the arms of Sleep herself.

I am open to the stillness of my soul.
This is where I long to be; this is where I now
go. My mind requests peace, my body seeks
release, and my heart whispers, "Please."
I am answered with deep sleep.

My soul is grounded in peace, free to sleep.

My bed is a safe haven for rejuvenation.

Relaxation breathes into me and I inhale
this serenity. Only qualities of love can pass
through my system. I rest in this sanctuary.
Healing sleep accompanies me, and now
it is safe to let everything else go.

All is well and
I am supported.

I don't need to figure everything out—
not all at once, and not tonight. My questions
are absorbed by the silence of night. I trust that
all I need will be revealed to me with perfect
clarity. For now, sleep is what's best.

Sleep is a salve
for my soul.

Sleep is coming to hold me together.
Every fearful, unloving illusion is replaced with
peace. My heart is being mended, and all my
pieces are being restored to wholeness.
As the struggles of today wash away,
I rest on the shores of harmony.

As I honor the innate wisdom of my body,
sleep happens naturally. I appreciate the gifts
my body is capable of giving. I accept the
natural intelligence I was born with,
and I let it guide the way.

*I am wholly capable
of falling asleep.*

I am worthy of the sleep I seek.

I am worthy of being restored back to
the vibrant health I knew when I was born.
I cast aside all doubt and free myself to receive
what my heart needs. I remember my highest
self, where worthiness is all that I know.

I am lifted higher than every darkened thought. As my body sinks into bed, I feel gravity pulling away all the heaviness from my day. Weights melt away and my mind settles into this silent place.

Every heavy thing falls away.

Sleep brings me home.

Ease is coming soon. Every breath
brings me closer to home. I am headed back
to the place where dreams are born, where
everything feels good. I am on my way home
again, with the moon as my steward.

I forgive this day.

I forgive myself for not wanting to forgive,
and I am willing to forgive everything that
comes after that. This day has been, and so
it also has an end. Forgiveness feels like
grace, and I feel myself falling into it.

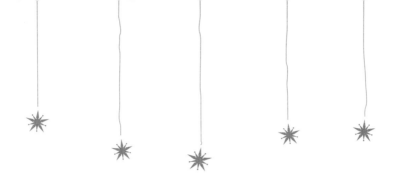

I ease into sleep with love all around me.

I am wrapped up in the arms of Love.
An easy energy begins to wash over my whole
body. I lie down in bed, trusting and thankful
for another chance to rest my head.

I welcome positive dreams.

As I focus on the beauty of life, dreams
come in to catch me. Everything softens now.
I am beckoned to the other side of awake.
I welcome this joyous, tranquil place.

I cherish my relationship with sleep.

Sleep is an ancient friend of mine.
I think of it kindly, with a mind quiet to all
other relationships. A soft smile crosses my
face because I know I am loved here. Sleep
reassures me with a goodnight kiss.

An easiness is in the air.

Peace trickles in with each belly breath,
filling me up with spaciousness. A sense of
quiet joy floats through me, a calm awareness
that subdues all worries. My brow softens.
Sleep comes easier to me now.

I believe in what's possible.

I embrace every ounce of my potential.
I don't need to see the whole path. When I must
adjust, I can. When I must let go, I can learn
how. I accept all good things that are
on their way now.

I am thankful for the chance to close my eyes.

I allow the healing energy of gratitude to pour from my heart. What a miracle it is to be alive, to breathe, to be still, to sleep. I feel blessed to be here—my blessings I hold dear.

My heart is
a harbor for love.

Only love is true and welcome in the harbor
of my heart. What is unloving does not stay and
humbly makes its way out to sea. Love alone
remains, safely held inside of me.

I honor my spiritual inheritance.
As I prepare for sleep tonight, I remember
how lovely it is to just *be*. Now I lay my body
down, this love and joy I keep, and I am brought
back to my homeland of peace.

Sleep is a conversation

with spirit.

There is no rush into the gifts of the night.

The darkness teaches me to trust that
everything can be a healing gift, all in due time.
I hold faithful certainty in my mind. I lie here
patient, knowing that I am going inward,
as surely as the stars shine.

I am safe right now.

"All is well" has been written on my heart.
I am safe in this space, enveloped in grace.
I know I am protected here, my wishes kept with
care. There is nothing right now that I need fear.

Everything I need to know is revealed
to me when it's for my greatest good.
The timeline and method are not mine to design.
The essence of what I desire is understood.
I release all outcomes and they dissolve into truth.

Sleep brings clarity.

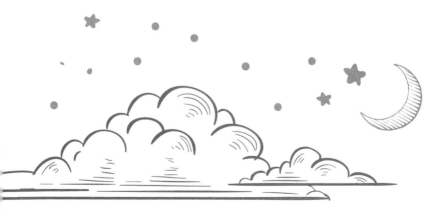

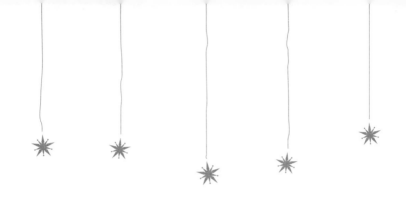

Loving kindness pervades my whole being.

I imagine the cleansing light of compassion
pouring through my whole body. It purifies and
corrects any deviance from love. I imagine this
soft light spreading from me to all beings. We
are all purified and made whole again with love.

This moment matters most.

The past has passed and the future has yet to be. This moment is the only moment where I can choose to be at peace with everything. I opt for a loving view of what has come before. Hope leads the way from here. I cherish the *now* even more.

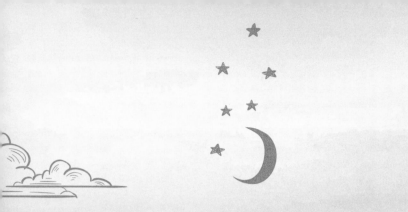

Each deep breath
is a love note.

I focus on slow, steady breathing.
Each breath feels like a drop of honey flowing
through me. Oxygen breathes ease into every
alcove of my body. My breathing is a
message of peace and harmony.

I return to my natural state of rest.

There's repose in my soul as I gather
my day and lay it down to sleep. A simple
memory of peace stays with me now. Comfort
is brought by the eve: I am allowed to unravel
and just *be* for a while.

I lie on a bed of roses.

Abundance and well-being are infinitely available to me. I rest my head and quiet my mind; freedom opens its gates for me. I may enter as I please. Trusting the potential of every dream, I am lulled to sleep by sweet possibility.

I entrust my body to sleep.

I bring my body into this bed and hand over all responsibilities. In sleep, all is working effortlessly. All pains and needs are met with great care. I trust that as I settle back down, my body regains entry to this state of loving repair.

Who I am is somehow more than I can fathom. I affirm a greater unity, and it awakens a fullness in my heart. There is nothing from which I am apart. I rest inside a great miracle, and I am grateful.

I rest, gratefully,
in the miracle of life.

My hopes are fulfilled in sleep.

I am not apart from what's right for me.
It is with certainty that this journey is meant
to be traveled by me. Hopes are brought to the
light. Errors are corrected as I sleep. There is
nothing I cannot do, have, or be.

Anything that doesn't feel good inside is allowed to breathe. There is nothing unworthy of the healing that sleep brings. A compassionate heart knows what I've been through. I am totally accepted. All worries are put to rest. Now, I can rest too.

I confide in sleep.

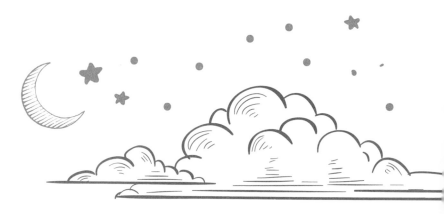

I receive the peace that's coming.

I feel every heavy thought being carried away now. Every block is fading away too. Whatever unease lingers in me is being changed with love. I am receiving the space I need to release the places that feel stuck. Peace fills me up.

I am an open channel for grace.

Grace greets me as I am. I am willing
to receive its gentle embrace. As I sink into
this forgiving place, all discord and resistance
are sent away. I am safe and sound.
It is okay for me to sleep now.

I am ready to heal.

Healing may not come in the form, or in the ways, I had planned for. Come what may, I walk the healing path. I value sleep and the role it plays in this part of my journey. I now accept the nourishment that sleep imparts.

Love is my guiding star.

I follow the guidance that love offers.
It locates my wounds and turns over all fear
and pain to the light. Love is my shepherd in the
night. Healing shines on me. I sink into sleep.
Love is the force that guides my way.

I don't need to push my thoughts away.
I relax and let peace come to me, filling every
thought with a lighter quality. This calming energy
sifts through my thoughts for me. My relaxation is
an invitation for peace to flow through me.

*Every thought is infused
with peace.*

I make peace with the unknown.

I don't need to know everything I think
I need to know—not right now. In this one simple
moment, sleep is the only thing that's calling for
me. Sleep is the answer and the way that
I honor what has yet to be.

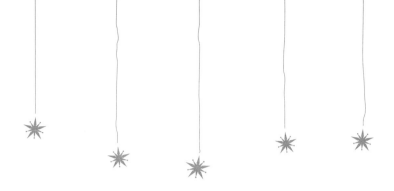

I am free to be in the present moment.

I am freed from the pull of yesterday, today, and tomorrow. The purity of this moment is where I'm meant to be. Every layer of me becomes lighter as I sink back into deep presence. This is my home.

It feels good to be still.

As I settle down in bed, my whole body sighs.
My breath rolls in and out like the tide. It's a
relief just to be here, alive. This still moment is
a gift—a waveless ocean, a breezeless sky.

Sleep is sewn into my soul.

The energy of serenity flows through my system. Healing light fills my veins. Every pained place in me is placed in Love's hands. I feel the threads of sleep as they are woven through all that I am.

Silence speaks

my name.

I pause and remember my true nature. The lull
of the night is the language of the spirit, the
companion of the heart. Everything I thought I was
cannot compare to the beauty of who I really am.
I am still and my soul remembers itself.

I am protected.

A deep ocean of sleep kindly covers the light
that I keep. My bedspread stretches out over me,
offering a safe space to lay my thoughts to sleep.
The moon shines away all shadows of doubt and
affirms that everything will be all right.

The stars call me home.

What a miracle that what makes the stars is also in me. Twinkling remnants of light continue to shine and I am comforted by their company. What a gift to sleep under the stars, always at home and never too far from where I long to be. There is stardust in my memory.

I am visited by beliefs that instill hope in my heart. Worries float behind and I keep loving alternatives close tonight. As I settle into a mindset of ease, it's only natural that sleep answers me.

I conjure up visions that feel good to me.

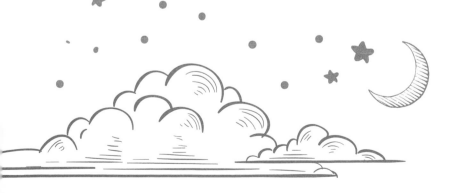

I am in the presence of sleep.

There's an unhurried quality in the air and in the room of my heart. Activity comes to a standstill. A friendly energy encircles me, cradling every wonder that could ever be. This is where I relax; this is when I sleep.

I am rooted in love. I am grounded in the earth. I am lowered into another depth of being. The soil feeds me and there is a calmness in the air that I breathe. Life loves me here and sleep greets me here. This is where I'll be tonight.

I sink into the natural world.

I welcome change.

Everything is always in transition. The present moment is home to limitless potential and all the wonder that I've yet to know. Nothing is possible without me being here. I welcome my transition into sleep, focusing on how grateful I am for what's coming into being.

Everything is in the process of being well.

Even while I sleep, the universe is working things out for my greatest good. I believe that an intelligence larger than me wishes only the best for my life on earth. This belief quiets the doubt inside my head, promising peace instead.

I am still, and I know.

I close my eyes and practice seeing with my heart. A gentle truth straightens out the kinks in my sight. I know that whatever I love cannot be apart from me. I know that everything will be okay and I am becoming free.

Where I am is okay.

I let go of all the fear that I should be somewhere other than here. There's no wrong decision, no path that I'm on that I'm not meant to be on. I swim in pure acceptance, receptive to every message. This is the right way.

The thoughts inside my head are not indicative of who I really am. I am more than their messages. I am the one who hears, who witnesses. What a relief: a thought is just a thought and not *me*.

I am more than the thoughts that happen to occur.

I forgive myself.

All is well in the house of my soul. All is well forevermore. Mistakes will one day be erased; until then, I'm graced by teachers of all kinds. I am here to evolve my consciousness. Every single experience is part of this divine process.

I am eternally enough.

I cannot be compared to anyone else,
for I am the only one who inhabits my
space. Just by being, I matter and I am
on purpose. In the eyes of eternity, I am
enough. I was born into this world enough.

Good things are meant for me. I am open to all
the ways the universe wants to bless me. Gifts
abound all around and are available to me as
I sleep. I feel good about life and I dream.

*I am open to receiving
what's meant for me.*

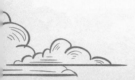

Sleep is my spiritual practice.

I am deeply involved with the practice of letting things be as they are. Sleep is a way of contacting my highest truth, my deepest heart. My journey becomes a state of absolute gratitude. I practice going there now.

I am drinking in this moment.

I am here, fully grateful for the gift of life that has been bestowed upon me. All my senses gather here. Time slows down in this place. I am wading in the moment, sinking deeper into it, sinking deeper into sleep.

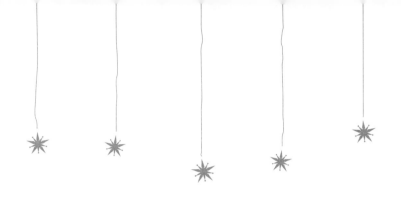

I am in tune

with nature.

My heart beats in harmony with the quiet
rhythm of the night. The moon composes a sweet
melody for me. I am in the sight of all things still.
All thoughts of separation leave. The one thing
I keep inside of me is unity.

I release all emotional negativity.

I loosen the bonds that chain me to a painful identity. I am not the pain that I feel. Negativity cannot define me. I accept what is here with me and untie myself from every illusion. I accept and release negativity in order to gain freedom.

Nothing is left undone.

Even as I sleep, life is being handled for me.
I may not know how to get everything done, but
I am willing to believe that, ultimately, nothing is
left undone. A higher order of things ensures
that everything is attended to.

Peace is my dwelling place.

My peace is becoming so deep, and so vast, that anything that is not peace disappears into it. I dwell in this open space; I disappear into it too. Everything becomes "no thing" here. Everything becomes a piece of eternity, endlessly at peace in itself.

I have all I need within me.
What I've yet to see will be shown to me
in the right light, time, and place. I am already
on the way there; I can rest here.

I am connected to

where I long to be.

I surrender for serenity.

I practice surrendering my worry, doubt,
and despair. I surrender every grievance.
I surrender everything so that it all
can be transformed while I sleep.

Some answers are found only in
the clear space of the here and now—
the moment with no questions. As I enter
this space, a different energy washes
over me. For now, sleep is my answer.

I welcome every answer
that sleep will give.

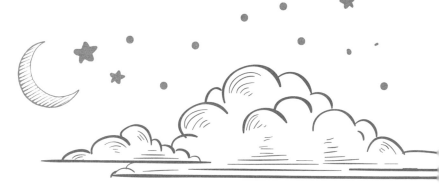

I resist nothing.

Every ounce of resistance is dissolved in
acceptance. I trust what comes and I hold on
to nothing. There is only freedom in my soul.
I am bound to no things and no thoughts.
I am as free as the wind that blows.

I am loved just for being.

It's easy to sleep knowing that I am loved at the core of my being. I do not judge the reasons why I am here: the universe makes no mistakes. The life I breathe is proof enough that love has a place in me.

Every thought passes through me with ease.

I am aware of the thoughts that pass through me and I let them pass through. All doors are open in my mind. Every thought is free to leave just as easily as it came because I pay it no mind.

I am comforted by visions of what I love.

I imagine my favorite place and I go there in my mind. I imagine what sights and sounds fill the air. I love being here. I take these visions to bed with me, and they take me to sleep.

There is no miracle too big or too small. As I focus on my love for sleep, all obstacles are withdrawn. I don't need to do anything but dwell in this loving state. My miracle starts to unfold immediately.

Sleep is a miracle that's available to me.

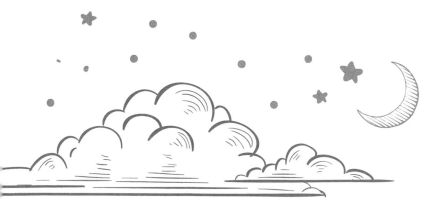

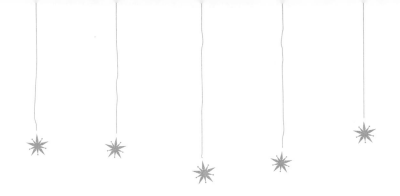

I can choose a thought that feels better.

No matter how fixed a thought pattern is,
I can choose again. Until another feel-
good thought sticks, I am willing to show up
and practice it. I am thankful for my simple
willingness: sleep is easier because of it.

Sleep is easy
for me tonight.

Where I was once doubtful, now I am hopeful.
My body listens to the current season I'm in
and a quiet knowing is prompted from within.
My rhythms are slow, patient, and wise.
Sleep is natural and I feel it beginning.

The past cannot hold me back.

By being present, I am released from the
past. I am free to lay all painful memories
aside now. I am free to let suffering rest for
a while. I cherish the times that carry love.
I carry only this love to sleep tonight.

I am eternally tied to my truth.

There's a place deep within me that remains unchanged. Here, I'm unaffected by the circumstances of my life and the happenings of my day. As I lie down to sleep tonight, I access this place. A new but ancient energy flows through me.

I have soil and stars in my soul. It is natural for me to always feel at home. I am connected to all things. The earth and sky together compose a lullaby, praising the part of me that is part of everything.

I am one

with everything.

I am willing to trust the process.

I am willing to trust the process of all
things, big and small, known and unknown.
I practice not needing to know, only needing
to trust that it's safe to waive control.

I accept the gift of a refreshed mind.

My mind slows. Mercy is delivered to every unconscious shadow. The cobwebs are cleared, the confusion enlightened. It's all sifted through for me, but not by me. I extend an invitation to sleep, asking for a little grace inside my head.

Forgiveness carries me to peace.

Forgiving thoughts replace bitter, sad, and guilty ones—I'm at least willing to try. As I move toward sleep, I consciously choose to keep only positive energy inside of me. Then there is peace. There is forgiveness in sight.

There is a time to shine and a time to rest.
There's time for all things, but not all at once.
I honor nature, who knows what's best. I feel
my own nature nodding in agreement.

*I am present enough
to cherish my cycles.*

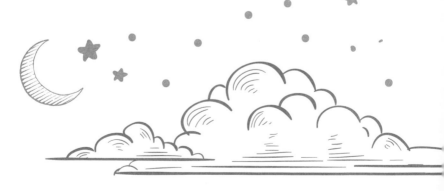

My only assignment is to trust.

Even and especially while I'm fast asleep—
though it seems like I'm doing nothing—the
constellation that is my life is being arranged for
growth. Healing is happening, filling me back
up. I trust that my only task right now is to trust.

I listen to my feelings as if they were good friends of mine. My pain is my guide. Every sensation I encounter inside is a messenger of healing. Every thought that feels good, or otherwise, wants me to realize how wonderful I can feel.

Every feeling is a friend.

I trust my body.

My body was born knowing how to sleep easily, naturally. How much this physical home of mine loves me; I now let it love me back to sleep. I close my eyes and everything else is taken care of for me.

I embrace being here.

I long to be fast asleep. Everything I accept turns into peace and takes me there. I hold on to this gratefulness for just being here, not needing to change a thing. There's a shift coming from the inside now and it takes me straight to sleep.

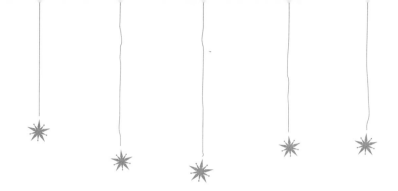

Energy is changing.

Life is a process of change. It's time for me to let my thoughts go to sleep. It's time for fresh, rejuvenating energy. I am ready for transformation. I am free from stagnation. It is time for something new.

I am unlimited.

Old, negative patterns do not bind me.
No amount of suffering can ever define me.
No label can describe the truths that live inside
me. This knowing brings me so much joy. Nothing
keeps me from sleeping soundly until the morning.

I forgive
and let go.

I forgive and let go as many times as
I need to. No matter my reasons for clinging
to painful seasons, I can go beyond them. I do
myself a favor, and I forgive and let go. I keep
nothing but peace for myself now.

I am wholly loving.

When I need assistance in letting go,
love comes to my side. At my core, love is all
I know. The essence of who I am holds no pain
inside. I am free and at peace. I fall asleep easily
tonight because love runs my life.

Sleep empowers me.

In my stillness I am strengthened. Every
waking dream basks in possibility while I sleep.
Restorative energy works its way through every
part of me. I honor the transition from thought to
peace. I am ready to be filled up again.

All problems have solutions.

Though I am confused now, I'll find clarity through sleep tonight. In the restful pause, space is made and clears the way for a brand new understanding. I move beyond what I don't yet know and trust that it will come to me when it's right.

I enter the chambers of sleep by allowing beautiful thoughts to cross my mind. Gratitude and patience displace any woes; all thoughts dissolve quickly into loving energy. The beauty I recall is a lullaby for my soul.

I let my mind dream beautiful things.

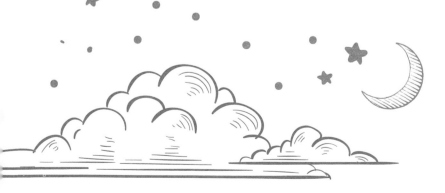

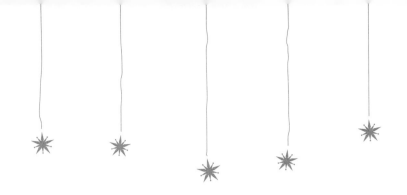

I can be easy on myself.

It is possible for me to give myself the courtesy of compassion. It is a practice, and I am willing to participate. Personal struggles are worthy of patience too. I am moving in a better direction now.

From this point forward, I am free from having to struggle. No fight; only faith. All I have to do is release and receive, as many times as I need to. Sleep, and all of life, is becoming much easier.

Everything is becoming easy for me.

My appreciation is a magnet for sleep.

I nourish a gratefulness that feels true in my heart.
I don't just think about it: I feel its soothing presence
touching every cell, altering my chemistry, and
making me well. My heartfelt appreciation is like
honey for the mind, body, and soul.

I am connected to
endless abundance.

There is an infinite pool of well-being
available to me always. I now choose to
tap into this boundless source of freedom.
With effortless ease, all the splendor of life
surrounds me and I am carried to sleep.

I don't believe in my negative thoughts.

I choose thoughts that align me with peace.
Any negative movement within is put to rest as
I settle in for the night ahead. I let the movement
naturally escape through my breath. Negativity
continues to release even while I'm asleep.

I let my perspective be corrected.

Whatever perspective is lingering from the day, I'm willing to have it transformed tonight. Something new wants to embrace me. I look forward to the nourishment I'm about to receive—I open my heart and close my eyes.

Every loving memory stays with me.
My heart is full with all of the wonderful
moments I hold dear. A kind energy rains upon
me, and it helps me forgive whatever needs
to be forgiven. Compassion settles in.

I fall asleep with kind thoughts and positive memories.

Everything I want also wants me.

I am worthy of the fulfillment of my
heart's desires. The essence of what I love
is its own reason for being. I look within and
I see that what I dream of having, doing,
and being also wants to experience me.

Sleep is my birthright.

It's okay for me to go to sleep. It's okay for me
to receive the replenishment I need to live the life
that's meant for me. I was born into this world on
purpose, and sleep is part of my journey.

Seeds of inner harmony lie dormant. I stop
seeking outside of myself and listen for their
song. They rejoice; they've been here all along.
I am present to receive what's already within me.
My presence delivers the gift of sleep tonight.

I am present with the potential of peace inside.

I hand over my worries to the moon.

I offer up any shadows to the light that's nearby. The moon shines away all fear, reminding me that I don't need to fight anymore. I surrender what's not mine to control. Now I can just *be*.

I make peace with time.

I am healing my relationship with time.
I don't look to the clock or calendar for the
meaning of my life. I let go of angst and allow
space for my heart's restoration. Savoring this
moment brings new meaning to my entire life.

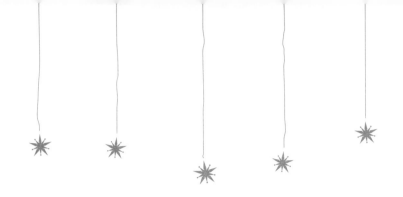

Sleep replenishes me.

I take a deep breath and realign myself with hope. Sleep lightens every burden, comforts all my woes. As the day is closing, I am opening up to an easier way of being. My cup is being filled. My mind is being emptied. My body is recovering.

My muscles are massaged while I sleep.

My weary body summons relief.
Sleep understands how to heal every tired
part of me. I unwind from life on earth and
mindfully release one muscle at a time. Gently,
limb by limb, sleep responds in kind.

I stick with love tonight.

Love is my highest potential, my deepest
truth, and my greatest accomplishment.
There is nothing that love cannot heal. Even
my incessant stream of thoughts is capable
of being healed with the presence of heart.
I focus on the essence of love right now.

As I inhale peace,
I exhale release.

Each inhale brings in rich, wholesome energy.
I inhale with presence and locate the areas that
crave release. I exhale mindfully, sending away
all tension and disease. Each exhale brings me
closer and closer to peace.

The darkness that surrounds me always
heeds the call of morning when it is time.
Right now, it is time to trust that every dusk
promises a dawn. I keep a light on in my heart,
honoring the dark, until the morning comes.

Every dusk has its dawn.

Hope is the energy that comforts me tonight.

I worry about nothing. Hope extends into the future so that I do not have to. Anxieties find their cure as I swim in silence and release all thinking. I drink in hopeful energy, sinking into sleep, accepting every form of healing.

I don't need to learn through pain anymore. I remember my lessons gladly tonight, grateful for the hidden gems they unearth. I honor life even when I do not understand it. I am ready for the next miracle that's in store for me.

I am ready to learn through joy.

I am understood.

I am free from my own separate little world.
I am willing to be part of something more
than I know. Every struggle I've ever known has
been known before and has been overcome with
devotion to something more. I am not alone.

Sleep is a pool of wisdom.

All things are part of an endless learning
process. My faith in what's possible is the
gateway to wisdom and knowledge. A higher
knowledge, deeper than the mind can go,
is accessible to my sleeping soul.

I give up all doubt.

I suspend my disbelief and choose to see through the eyes of certainty. I am sure of the miracles that are now being drawn to me. I am receptive to their messages, relaxed and ready to be free of doubt. I am not without support.

There is only room
for gratitude.

I leave no space for unhappiness to dwell
in me. As my heart pumps gratitude into every
cell of my body, I'm filled with awe. I am grateful
for the sweetness that's flowing through me.
I am ready to follow the call of sleep.

My favorite sounds from life on earth
form a melody inside my heart. I am carried
by their songs into the dark and dreaming
night. I fly easily toward sleep; the sounds
are my wings. As I listen to their lullabies,
they become my dreams.

I imagine soothing sounds

carrying me to sleep.

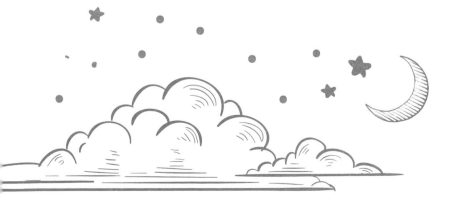

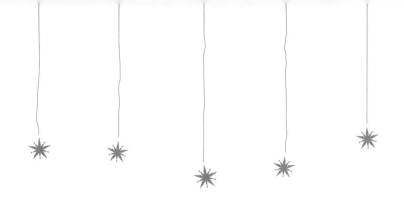

Sleep bestows its gifts upon me.

A gentle rain washes away all attachments
to today. The gift of grace awaits my stay
tonight, and I accept its invitation. I am grateful
for the blessings that are reserved for me,
knowing full well that I am on my way.

It's good
to feel good.

I am growing comfortable in a state of joy
and trust. I am harmonizing with the natural
energy flow of life. I don't rely on fear for a sense
of who I am anymore. I accept my worthiness
and welcome happiness forevermore.

I am grounded.

As I lie down for sleep, I envision every inch of
my body sinking into my bed. I feel myself being
pulled into the ground, gently and steadily. Today's
experiences are being released as I sink. Slowly,
each cell finds itself being drawn into sleep.

I am becoming who I am meant to be.

Sleep nurtures my journey to my highest self. I am given the nourishment I need to continue my exploration of who I can be. Aiding every meaningful path I could ever wish to explore, sleep takes care of me.

One breath at a time will soothe my mind. There is no rush, only the hush of hope. I am open to receiving the sleep my body needs, and sleep encourages me to just keep breathing.

Sleep comes one breath at a time.

Sleep has a home in me.

Pockets of peace expand throughout my
body. Here, sleep settles in comfortably. Cozy
and safe, there is room enough for a full night's
sleep to stay. I treasure all the places inside
of me that are home from dusk till dawn.

I trade resistance

for an invitation.

I dissolve the fear of not having, doing,
or being enough. I tune in to the energy of love.
I don't push or pull; I let the universe catch
up with my dreams. My faithful presence
invites the peace that wants to guide me.

130

I set everything free.

I feel the sweet release of night swirl
around me, holding and unfolding all of my
fears. Every unworthy, unhealthy, and unloving
feeling is healing. It is becoming easier to let go
and rest in the glow of the night that's here.

Every fall I take is a prayer for forgiveness. Every detour into fear is a call for the love that's missing. As soon as I am ready to receive my own forgiveness, I am free. I reminisce about the love I still have to give.

I am draped in forgiveness.

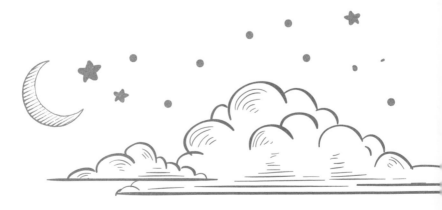

I try trusting instead.

I am free from every "why" and "how." I play
with the idea that everything is okay right now;
it is well in the journey and in the end. I release
"should" altogether. I choose peace instead,
trusting that I am okay in the flow.

At this very moment in time life is lining up so much beauty for me to see. I don't need to know the details of how this beauty will arrive because I'm certain it will be something incredible. I close my eyes. Every blessing is on schedule.

Life showers me with goodness.

Love never ends.

Everything loving is true, and what is unloving
is only a temporary illusion. Fear, hurt, and
heartbreak eventually go back to love, and so do I.
Every ounce of love I have ever given and received
is kept for me. Nothing I love can ever die.

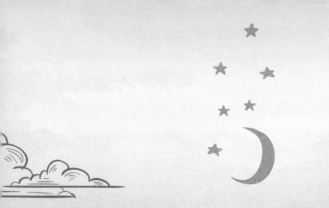

I fall asleep with imagery of the universe.

I imagine every awe-inspiring nook and cranny of the universe. How vast life is. How miraculous that I am alive to contemplate this. I am a witness to even the smallest miracles, which is a profound gift.

I rest inside a pause.

Between today and tomorrow a certain
calmness rules my world. I stop spinning and
my soul thanks me for this breathing space. This
pause is ready to take me in, ready to show me
how everything is nourished, one breath at a time.

I am gentle with myself.

I choose to believe that everything is a
call to love a little more. I choose to open my
doors inward and call myself a friend. I stop
keeping score. The love I dream about tonight
is the love I'm now bringing forth.

I plant a positive seed.

I can think of one thought that feels good to me. As I head for sleep, I plant this seed of positivity. The energy of this thought lingers in my body, planted in fertile soil, spreading its roots deeper into my truth as I sleep.

I see myself in perfect health.

I spend this moment visualizing perfect health inside of me. Every tiny cell is bathed in healing light. This radiance fills me up from the inside out, preparing me for a full night's sleep. The stars that shine inside of me heal me as I dream.

I offer thanks.

I am thankful for the roof over my head and the pillow underneath my head. I realize there are many things to be thankful for and they don't have to be big things. I find one thing to whisper "thank you" to, and what I love is given wings.

I breathe myself
back to calm.

Every time my mind gets carried away,
I bring myself back to my breath. I force nothing.
I picture each inhale carrying me inward
and each exhale taking a thought with it.
One breath at a time, I calm the world within.

142

I know what really matters when
I stop to appreciate. I know who I am when
I stop trying to be something else. My worth
does not depreciate based on any opinion.
My truth remains unchanged by what has
been done. I am forever at home.

I remember who I am.

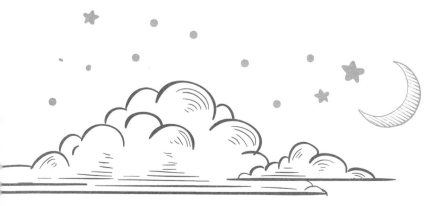

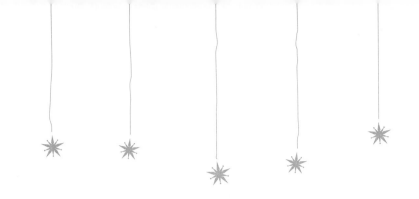

I am loved,
and I Am Love.

Love is closer to who I am than any name,
label, or form I've picked up along the way.
I cannot lose something that I am. As the day
fades away, this message vibrates in me:
I am loved, and I Am Love.

My highest good is supported and every request is understood. My wishes are fulfilled without a doubt as I relax and let myself return to love. There is nothing left to keep me up tonight because all is right and well inside.

Everything happens for me.

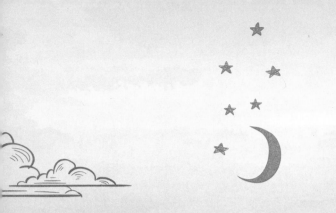

Peaceful energy is growing within.

I feel the mental chatter leave because
it has no place to stay inside of me. This chatter
is not mine to keep. I hold a positive empty space
in my mind. This feeling of peace expands
and brings me to sleep.

Sleep is my medicine.

I don't need to fix everything; all I need
is sleep. I don't need to save and conquer;
I need to let the love in. There are many cures
for many things, but tonight sleep is my
best medicine. I let this truth sink in.

I choose comfortable thoughts.

I opt for thoughts that feel comfortable tonight. I align myself with peace. I carve a pathway to all desired things, people, and experiences with every comfortable thought I think. Comfort becomes my state of being and brings me right to where I want to be.

I am here to live a wonderful life.

My only task is to live my life as openly and truly as I can. I let this moment fill me up, and I choose to let all the wonder in. Tomorrow is another chance to live fully, to try again.

My heart is still beating after another day;
I made it to tonight. I am loved and cared for—
all day long and every night. I don't need
to fight with what happens internally;
my heart wants the best for me.

I sign a peace treaty

with my heart.

I am free tonight.

I am free from the demands of
judgment and am gifted a little grace in its
place. The requests of regret dissolve tonight.
All nagging thoughts are removed from my head
until there's no trace of them in sight. I count my
blessings and say goodnight.

I am grateful to be alive.

To be here on this blue and green planet
is such a precious gift. I breathe in oxygen
without thinking twice. My heart beats minute
after minute. I am blessed to know the ebb and
flow of life; the earth is a friend of mine.

I fall asleep with a dream.

There is a dream that I keep close to my heart.
This dream is part of who I am. Every peaceful
vision feeds me hope and lets me know that I am
capable. I let this hope support all that I am.

What I need is surely coming to me. There is enough life available for everything; what was once lost becomes a foundation for something more. I let this perspective sink in overnight. The energy I embrace makes me a magnet for more.

In sleep,

I attract what I need.

Relief is never too far away.

At any given moment I am just a few
deep breaths away from feeling better.
Right now, I am just a few deep breaths away
from feeling the relief that I crave. Nothing
that replenishes me is ever too far away.

I believe in the possibility of something new.
I can make happy new memories and extract
love from what I've been through. There is hope
for me here and something to look forward to.
I'm open to the good that's coming through.

I believe in a

better tomorrow.

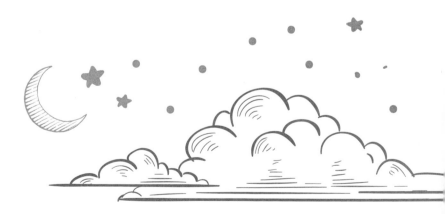

I sleep in pure positive energy.

As I fall asleep, I'm truly falling into pure positive energy. Every moment that I spend asleep is a moment spent in perfect harmony. Every part of me loves everything about this place. I imagine entering this supremely happy state.

I prioritize love tonight.

The deeper I decide to love, the better
I feel—no matter what. I choose to rest in love
tonight because the deepest parts of me know
that it's what I need. Love above all else:
this is my highest priority.

Sleep is a sacred ritual.

I honor the natural rhythms of my body
and cherish the day as it turns to night. My
body knows what to do; I can trust in this deep-
seated insight. Starlit skies call me back to
sleep. I settle into my divine birthright.

I am alive in my body, at home in this moment. Trillions of cells know me by heart and want me to live. My heart beats faithfully. I am filled with gratitude for this gift. Every cell is grateful.

I am at home in the present moment.

I dwell in possibility.

As I sit in the present moment, possibility expands in every direction. I can alter the vibration of my past and set a new vibration for the future. I am powerful here. I am peaceful now. Even sleep comes easily in my presence.

Sleep is in the stars for me.

Sleep promises itself to a mind at ease.
I now affirm that I am free from everything
and all tensions continue to leave. My energy
gradually matches the energy of sleep. I welcome
a smooth transition from awake to dreaming.

I am free to believe in what feels loving to me.

My truth is not limited to any one belief.
A belief is just a thought pattern, and a thought
can be changed. I am not stuck in anything that
makes me feel less than loved and loving.

I stop spinning and let the world spin without me. There's so much peace right here, and I'm so glad that I'm stopping to feel it. It's been here all along. I decide to stay here all night long, in this song of peace.

I choose peace now.

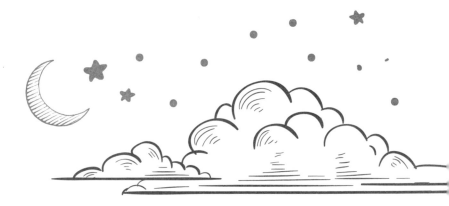

I am making space.

In the realm of sleep, space is made for me to live with more ease. I don't waste time; I make space. I don't lose opportunity; I make space for something completely new. I am not defined by the confines of time. I am spacious.

I am light enough for sleep to carry me.

My journey into sleep is all about releasing what I don't need. The less I carry, the lighter I become. I don't add to myself; I lighten my load. Every burden I drop makes it easier for sleep to carry me home.

I don't need to control my thoughts and they don't need to control me. I welcome a truce and choose peace above everything else. I let my mind be. I give it room to think and breathe. We are friends. We can both go to sleep.

My mind is my friend.

I experience love.

Anything that I don't want leaves my experience. I hold a space for the joy that emerges from within. I remember how it feels to inhabit only love, to breathe only life. This is the memory I fall asleep with tonight.

Feeling good brings me home.

I don't need anyone's permission to feel
good about myself—I only need my own. I allow
myself to be as I am and acceptance takes me
home again. There is peace in my mind, freedom
in my body, and rest in my soul.

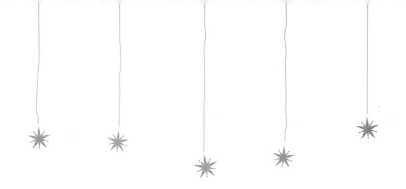

I listen to my intuition.

The inspiration I seek rests within. I am silent and
I listen to what my intuition has to say. I listen
with my breath; I see with my heart. I'm learning
to feel my way back to the wisdom inside of me.

I follow the moon

to sleep.

I keep in my mind's eye a vision of the night sky.
Soft and patient, the moon is my lamp that guides
the way back. I follow its glow all the way home.
I am on the right track. I know where I'm going.

I am everything.

I am vulnerable and I am strong. I am fearless
because all my fears reroute to love. There are
dark skies in me and there are stars that shine
until the sun comes up. I am many things and
I am no thing. I am everything all rolled into one.

I believe in the healing power of sleep.

Sleep heals me on every level—mental, emotional, physical, spiritual. The night provides ample nourishment and clarity. Everything my heart, head, body, and soul need is graciously given to me. I trust the guidance I receive while I'm asleep.

I am connected to everything and everyone
I have ever loved and have ever received love
from. I am tethered to every blessing of the past
and all those yet to come. My cells radiate all the
joy I've ever known and will ever know.

I am connected to

all good things.

I am the ruler of my own skies.

I decide how loving I feel inside. My self-worth is not tied to what happens. I allow myself to be who I am and to not feel "less than." I am devoted to my inner world. I am a friend to myself.

I imagine what my dreams feel like as
they come to fruition in everyday life. I focus on
the energy of the beautiful things I'm imagining.
I set the intention to bask in the glow of joy
tonight and I let the dream take flight.

I summon my dreams.

My awareness is expansive.

I explore a state of awareness that is always unfolding in every direction. All the sections of my life are pieces of a bigger mystery. I close my eyes and imagine more than what I know life to be. I close my eyes and dream.

I swim in the steady stream of life.

I go with the flow, floating easily in this season of my life. I don't cling to anything outside of who I am for my peace of mind. Everything I need for a full and happy life is right here, now—inside.

Surrender feels good to me.

I surrender all doubt, for the light of
morning brings new hope. For now, the night
offers me another chance to release. I make an
offering of peace. There is an understanding
between life and me, and I relax into sleep.

I give myself a break.

I forgive myself for ever having trouble falling
asleep. I see the detours into frustration and lace
them with present-moment peace. In this moment,
I accept my nonpeace and it turns into peace.
I feed every reason why I'm worthy of sleep.

My inner world is balanced and clear.

With each breath I take, inner peace replaces turmoil. All the clutter melts away. Chaos slowly disappears and comfort takes its place. Attachments fade and fear loses its hold on me. My inner world is a beautiful place to be.

I glow like the moon outside my window.
All the energies that live inside of me are seen
and soothed. My vibration is raised through
the power of love, the light that transcends
all others. I am soft and steady and renewed
by the light of the moon.

I am luminous.

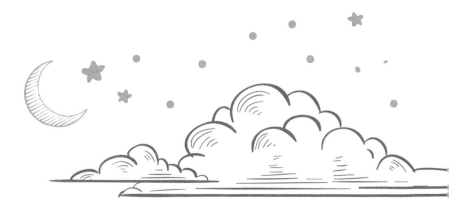

I breathe away the day.

My breathing is like slow, rolling waves.
Clear waters purify my veins, washing away
the debris from today. All the aches and worries
inside of me are carried in the current and
swept out to sea. My breath carries me
to sleep, and I am grateful.

Dear universe:

I am thankful.

I send a love note to the universe: Thank you for letting me know what it's like to live. I'm truly blessed, even when there's suffering. If I can't take anymore, I will try to give. I appreciate another chance to open my heart and live.

External chaos cannot get to me. I give myself
more credibility than I give the disturbances
outside of me. I believe in my capacity for sound
sleep regardless of any noise surrounding me.
I can sleep, no matter what happens to be.

I can sleep,

no matter what.

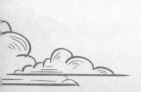

I release

blocked emotions.

Sleep heals every uncomfortable emotion that
has found a hiding place in me. I open myself to
transformation and a deep reservoir of healing
becomes available to me. I now place my attention
on something that feels easy, comforting,
beautiful, or hopeful. I feel the release.

I am present in my body.

I focus on the uncomfortable or pained places in me. I imagine sending peaceful, aware energy there, one breath at a time. A gentle hum takes over; all my cells begin to vibrate ever so slightly, radiating relief. My peace grows deep.

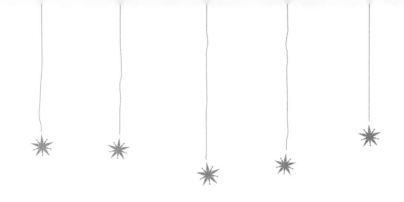

I am in the stillness
of a beautiful room.

My fulfillment rests in the eternal *now*, which
is where I rest tonight. There is no struggle
required of me. I am soothed by the composition
of peace pouring through me. It's beautiful here,
in the comfort of this room.

I am at peace.

I let go of the struggle. I surrender to ease.
Life is peaceful and calm as I prepare for a full
night's sleep. I am surrounded by well-wishes.
I feel the love raining down. Life is on my side
tonight. It's time for sleep now.

I imagine oneness.

I breathe in deeply and my mind comes home to my body. I breathe again and I imagine that I am closer to everything than I could ever know. Where I once believed in separation, I am now shown something new and something old: everything is in union.

I let everything be so that I can sleep.

I am willing to let things be as they are, knowing that nothing is ever too far from transformation. All the information that feels stuck inside is carefully filtered through sleep tonight. Every ounce of resistance fades and I am changed.

Gentle showers of gratitude sprout seeds of loving awareness. I till the soil with hope and breathe in fresh air. As each petal of sleep unfolds, the wisdom of my body harvests the beauty of my soul.

My soul is a garden that I tend with care.

I follow my inner compass.

I am not the streams of thought inside my head;
I am the observer of all thoughts, the clarity
underneath confusion and chaos. I tune in to the
awareness that speaks from my soul. I listen to
the still, small voice within. I am home again.

Sleep is the most healing period of
my day. I experience the weightlessness
of aligning with this calm and centered place.
Every phase of sleep contributes to my inner
peace and total well-being. Naturally, easily,
I yield to the wishes of sleep.

*Sleep is my
healing partner.*

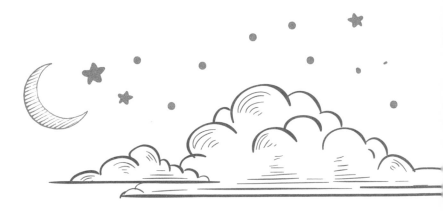

I am floating
in freedom.

I experience total inner fulfillment as I rest
inside the present moment. Here, I am beyond
the reach of anything and everything outside
of the *now*. I reach beyond the horizon of
any burdensome beliefs. My truth is
measureless, precious, and free.

I care about my well-being.

I am a friend to myself, which makes me
a better friend to everyone else. I treasure
the love I'm capable of experiencing. I give
myself space to nurture my strengths. There's
an abundance of support available to me
because I care about myself.

I am loving myself to sleep.

I let go of any limiting beliefs. I am willing
to accept myself completely. I practice
believing that I am already whole, already
full of the love I wish to know. I am loved and
loving. I am enough, right here and now.

I am connected to miracles.

If there's magic in this world, sleep is the portal through which I know it. My mindset and whole being experience subtle and sudden shifts—what feels like magic is my miracle. Sleep is the ultimate soul elixir and I'm drinking that sweet relief tonight.

I am healing.

Healing is my present-moment reality. I'm not just on the healing path now; I have become the path. I am healing and I Am Healing. From my fingertips to my toes and to the depths of my mind, heart, and soul, healing is part of me.

Sleep fertilizes my core desired feelings. I am enriched and empowered to feel the way I want to feel. I visualize the roots of every single dream finding their place inside of me—inside of sleep. I'm closer to my own freedom.

I start to feel like my best self.

I transcend all fear.

There is nothing that the essence of love is not
capable of correcting. In my heart of hearts, I am
eternally okay. My loving core ensures that I rise
higher than every fear. Through lessons and light
I am brought closer to the peace that's here.

I am made strong through sleep.

Tomorrow's tasks are made easier with a full night's sleep tonight. The strength I receive helps me to be a gentle force of inspiration in my world. I access calm, clarity, and creativity while my brain, body, and heart recharge.

I live a fluid journey. As I breathe in the
depth of this moment, the pressure of time is
lifted. I am alive, in the *now* and outside of time.
I am fluid. I become boundless as I drift into
sleep, tied to nothing and totally free.

I am timeless.

I let the universe arrange life for me.

I allow myself the freedom to be supported
by a universal plan. I force nothing and make
no demands. I bathe in a wide emptiness beyond
any understanding. Life is so much easier now
that I've let love take the reins.

I am an energetic
match for sleep.

The moon showers me with healing. The night
blankets me with care. I am offered gentle guidance
from above, wrapped in warmth and cradled with
feelings of hope. The energy I radiate follows the
moon into the night with full trust.

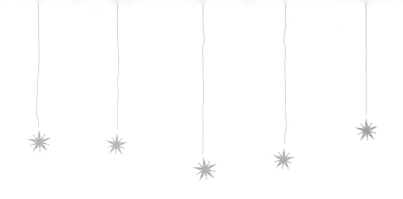

I am opening every door to sleep.

I am deeply connected to my dreams when I am open to the reprieve that sleep brings. I swing the door of my heart wide open and welcome the downtime I need. I make an offering. I make a connection with sleep.

I declare peace.

Peace is my ultimate home. My heart beats in a
rhythm so slow. Truth sweeps through and I relax
into the breath of life. I am homeward bound, for
I have found home in the depth of this still night.

about the author

JENNIFER WILLIAMSON is the author behind AimHappy.com, a blog devoted to the joy that can be found in healing. Rising from the ashes of losing her brother to suicide, she sparks daily loving communication on her website and social media platforms through positive poetry, uplifting affirmations, quotable curations, and down-to-earth wisdom. Every composition is a gentle force of inspiration, offering replenishment for the depleted, hope for the desperate, and love for those who have forgotten. Born and raised in the beautiful countryside of New England, she currently enjoys lakeside living in Central Massachusetts.